HOW TO PASS A MARIJUANA DRUG TEST

PROVEN METHODS TO FOOL YOUR BOSS AND BEAT THE SYSTEM

I0463770

By Simon Stone

ISBN-13: 978-1500809027

ISBN-10: 1500809020

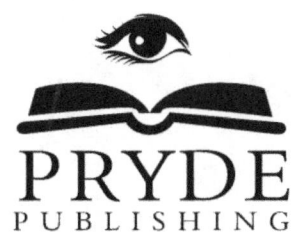

PRYDE
PUBLISHING

WHY I WROTE THIS BOOK

I want to congratulate you for getting the book, *"How to Pass a Marijuana Drug Test: Proven Methods to Fool Your Boss and Beat the System"*. Do you need to fool your boss or beat the system? Then this book is for you! Having personally dealt with drug tests on many occasions, I have scoured libraries and the internet for solutions to this problem. There is a lot of misinformation out there and I know what it's like to fail a drug test because of bad advice. There are not many books on the subject and the books that do exist are either outdated, misinformed, or don't contain enough useful tips and information to actually help you pass a drug test. Therefore, I have collected the most current solutions and information for this problem into a single book.

I don't like to make outrageous claims but I do believe this book is possibly the most definitive guide currently on the market dealing with marijuana drug tests. Best of all, I am offering it at an affordable price so that this information can reach as many people as possible. I do this because I passionately believe that marijuana drug tests are unnecessary and invasive. Please recommend this book or share it with your friends. If you enjoyed this book, also be sure to leave a review on Amazon. This book offers the most up-to-date information about drug tests and the most current solutions to pass them. You will learn:

- The science behind urine, saliva, blood, and hair follicle drug tests and how your knowledge of this science can help you beat drug testing procedures.

- The factors that will increase your chances of passing a drug test.

- Methods and strategies to pass any type of drug test 99% of the time and the concrete scientific reasons that these methods work.

- The factors that will increase your chances of passing a drug test.

- And many other valuable tips and information to help you stay one step ahead of the Man.

I want to extend my thanks to you once again for getting this book. I hope you enjoy it!

TABLE OF CONTENTS

NOTE FROM THE PUBLISHER

Pryde Publishing is dedicated to bringing readers informative, inspirational, and innovative books on a variety of different subjects. We are truly grateful to our authors for producing high-quality work and we are proud to deliver their material to our audiences. To contact our authors, discuss their books or stay updated on the latest releases, please follow us on our social media pages:

Facebook: facebook.com/PrydePublishing

Twitter: twitter.com/PrydePublishing.

We frequently promote our new releases by offering the books *completely free of charge* for a limited time. Make sure that you follow these pages so that you do not miss out on our great offers.

MARIJUANA AND DRUG TESTS: THE HISTORY AND THE SCIENCE

Marijuana—it's possibly the most popular illicit drug in the world and probably safer than that cup of coffee you drink every morning to drag yourself to work. Most sane people in the new century realize this for what it is: irrational and stupid. To understand the contradiction you have to go back to the beginning of 20th century America. Although the scope of this book does not permit us to go into detail on the subject, I will briefly touch upon it for the benefit of those who may be curious. At the beginning of the 20th century, when America was on its way to greatness, traditional colonialism was in its death throes. Capitalism was booming, empires were in decline, and America was about to take its place as one of the only superpowers on the planet.

America often prides itself as being a nation of immigrants—and with good reason. America's rising status as a superpower came about through the hard work of the American people. But they encountered a problem; namely, there was a lot of work and not enough workers. People flocked to the United States from around the world in search of a better life and to get their own piece of the American Dream. This solved the problem of America's labor shortage but it gave rise to a host of other problems. The nation had only recently abolished slavery through a painful civil war; racism was still rife; and the Civil Rights Movement was not to come for several decades.

In periods of economic depression when work dried up it was easy to blame recent immigrants for their problems, particularly Asians, Blacks, and Mexicans. They were viewed as job stealers but, as America began to forge its national identity and culture, foreign habits and customs were becoming unwelcome. Outsiders are typically identified by broad, general features that they may share in common. Things like hairstyle, clothing, skin color, and so on, become identifying features to categorize outsiders. In a similar manner, drugs became one way of identifying outsiders. Asians were associated with opium; Mexicans with cannabis; and, despite being more popular with white middle-class women at the time, blacks were associated with cocaine.

It is not hard to see then how this paved the way for the prohibition of marijuana and the War on Drugs. This also ensured employers that their workers would be productive. Employers want their workers to take drug tests not because they are concerned about their health but because they want obedient, productive workers that are going to make them as much money as possible. The government even attempted to outlaw alcohol at one point but this obviously proved to be unpopular and the campaign ended as a miserable failure—not to mention, the law was essentially ignored by the upper-class since it was primarily aimed at the working and lower class. So the next time you're standing in a toilet cubicle peeing into a cup for your employer, just remember that a century of history, politics, economics and racism has led up to this moment.

The unfortunate thing about marijuana is that it stays in your system for so long. You would have to be an idiot of the worst kind to fail a cocaine drug test since it only stays in your system for 24 hours or, at most, 48 to 72 hours for chronic abusers. By contrast, it can take your body a whopping 30 days or more to pass a urine test for marijuana. On the other hand, this is also what makes marijuana one of the least addictive drugs—since it lingers in your system for so goddamn long your body does not experience cravings and withdrawal symptoms on the same level as a coke or heroin user, for example. This is because of a little something known as science.

However, the more you smoke the longer it will stay in your system and vice versa. This is an important principle to remember but depending on which method you choose from this book to pass your drug test, you could feasibly smoke a huge bowl a minute before the test and still pass (by the way, I do not recommend this!). It goes without saying then that if you tried marijuana for the first time only a week ago and you're worried about testing positive for a urine test tomorrow you probably don't have much to worry about. You should also be aware that there are different types of drug tests. These can include urine, saliva, blood and hair follicle tests. All of these have different detection rates *and* different detection time frames, which will be covered in more detail in later chapters. Urine drug tests are by far the most popular test to use since they are relatively straightforward, reliable, and inexpensive.

Why does cannabis remain in the body for so long, I hear you ask? To understand this you have to understand the mechanics of tetrahydrocannabinol, or THC for short. THC is the main active ingredient in marijuana that induces the high we all know and love by binding to cannabinoid receptors in the body. THC fits into these receptors like a key fits into a lock. So why do we have cannabinoid receptors? Our body naturally produces cannabinoids, such as anandamide. In other words, by smoking cannabis we are mimicking a process that naturally occurs within the body already. Women out there might find this comparable to the hormone estrogen. When estrogen levels drop during menopause, some women supplement this by taking in estrogen from other sources such as soy or yams or even synthetic estrogen from pharmaceutical products.

THC accumulates in the body by clinging to fat. If you've ever tried to cook cannabis into an edible form you would probably know that it has to be done by using a fat-containing ingredient such as butter or olive oil. Marijuana is fat soluble but not water soluble. This is why trying to make weed tea is a waste of good weed unless you add something like full fat milk or butter into the mix. As your body burns fat for energy, THC is released into the bloodstream. Therefore, the less fat you have the easier it is to pass a drug test since THC has less fat to cling on to in the first place and THC accumulation will be lower than someone with more fat. Less body fat is probably also an indication of having a fast metabolism, meaning that your body is burning fat, and thus THC, at a more rapid rate. This relationship between THC and fat is the reason that it stays in the body for longer periods than other drugs and why marijuana withdrawal symptoms are either minimal or non-existent for most people; it exits the body at a slower pace.

Different strains and preparations of marijuana will have different concentrations of THC, which can affect the length of time it takes to pass a drug test. Urine tests are looking for the presence of THC in your system or, more specifically, THC-COOH—a metabolite that is produced when the liver breaks down THC. THC-COOH can be detected for much longer periods of time than THC because THC is metabolized into this form at a faster rate than THC-COOH can exit the body. 50 ng/mL is the most common cutoff level that drug screening companies are using when testing for THC-COOH. Less common cutoff thresholds are 20 and 100 ng/mL. Blood and saliva tests generally look for the presence of actual THC rather than its metabolite form THC-COOH. This is the reason for their lower time frames of detection, because THC is broken down rapidly into metabolites. So whereas urine tests can detect marijuana for 30 days or more, a saliva test can only detect it for a period of about 1-3 days at most.

To summarize, you must take several things into consideration when taking a drug test. In no certain order, these are:

- THC amount: the amount, type and/or preparation of marijuana you are using can affect the time it will take to pass a drug test.

- Body fat: THC binds with fat cells. The more body fat you have, the more THC will have accumulated and the longer it will take for the THC to exit your body.

- Frequency of use: light users will pass a drug test faster than a heavy user.

- Type of test: different tests have different rates of detection and different detection time frames.

So, are you ready to beat that drug test? I hear you, let's get started.

URINE TESTS I: FOUR PROVEN METHODS

I have listed below the average time frames that various types of smokers may appear positive for marijuana on a urine test:

- One Time Users: 1-6 days

- Moderate Users: 7-13 days

- Frequent Users: 15+ days

- Heavy Users: 30+ days

Please remember that these time frames are only valid if you *have not consumed* anything during that period. For example, if you're a moderate user with a test coming up in 10 days and you smoke a bowl the day before your test you will probably show up positive. So don't do anything stupid! Although, as I have already mentioned, you could feasibly do this with some of the methods you will learn here but it's always best to play it safe and stop smoking for a while. If you can simply stop smoking for 30 days then do it because it's the easiest solution in this situation. Some very heavy smokers have reported showing positive for 45-90 days after quitting. This is relatively rare and most users should not be worried about being positive for this length of time unless they have spent every waking moment smoking the green. Even if you are this type of person you have nothing to worry about with this book in your hands. Having said that, let's get on with it.

METHOD 1: EXERCISE, DIET, AND ABSTENTION

If you find out that you have a drug test coming up, the best thing to do is immediately stop consuming marijuana. This is a common sense approach that should be followed no matter what kind of test is being used. If you have enough time to prepare for the drug test, this is the best path to take. Depending on what kind of marijuana consumer you are, the time it will take to produce clean urine will vary. Use the guide on time frames above to get an estimate. In addition, there are a few other things you can do to cut this time frame down considerably.

As you should already know by now, THC is stored in the fatty tissues of your body. To improve your chances of passing a test you have to get rid of the THC metabolites stored in your fat by burning it as energy. So how do we do this? With some good old-fashioned diet and exercise. Your metabolism indicates how fast energy is used and it can come from both sugar and fat. You'll need to raise your metabolism and eat a low-sugar diet because, if given the option, your body will burn sugar for energy before it burns fat. But in this case we want our body to be using fat as its energy source to get rid of the THC metabolites. There is no shortcut to raise your metabolism. However, there are some things that will help.

Each time you eat, your metabolic rate rises. Instead of eating 3 large meals you'll want to eat 5 or 6 smaller meals spread throughout the day. Breakfast is the most important because it jumpstarts your metabolism. The other important key to raising your metabolic rate is exercise. This raises your metabolism higher than normal and kicks it into high gear. With exercise, both aerobic and anaerobic exercises are equally as important. Aerobic exercise will burn THC-containing fat and anaerobic exercises increase muscle mass—and an increase in muscle leads to an increase in your metabolic rate. This combination of diet and exercise is something we should all do anyway but for those who don't usually follow a strict diet or exercise you'll want to do this right up until the day of testing.

On the day of your drug test I recommend fasting because you want your metabolism to be as low as possible so that any remaining THC metabolites aren't running wild throughout your body. You'll also want to be using sugar as your energy source so drink some juice or anything with high sugar content because if fat is burned it's going to release metabolites into your urine. This step isn't completely necessary and you could probably take a rest from all your hard work but it might be a good idea if you want to be cautious. Make sure you pee at least once before going in to do the test because the first pee of the day contains the most metabolites.

When you go in to give your urine sample, take it "midstream". This means peeing into the toilet for a little and then taking a sample from the middle of your urination. This gives you the best chance of providing urine with a low concentration of metabolites. End your pee by aiming back into the toilet. Sometimes you'll be asked not to flush so that they can confirm the sample you have provided is actually urine and is the same color—so make sure you follow their instructions.

METHOD 2: DILUTION

There was once a time when you could simply drink a ton of water and dilute your urine to make the concentration of metabolites negligible. This made passing a drug test relatively simple. But when labs started to catch on to this they started analyzing things such as creatinine levels, specific gravity, and the color of the urine. The dilution method began to fall out of favor when this started to happen. However, dilution can still work so long as you follow some additional steps. The best thing about the dilution method is that it can be performed on relatively short notice and no diet or exercise is necessary.

Creatinine is a chemical waste product that is produced by the breakdown of the creatine in your muscles. Kidneys filter this from your blood and it exits the body through your urine. However, creatine can be taken into the body from other sources. Athletes often use creatine supplements and begin their supplementation with a "loading phase". This is typically 20g for about 5 days and then 5g for each day following the loading phase. Creatine supplements are available at places like GNC. Another great source of creatine is red meat. Creatine takes around 24 hours to metabolize into creatinine but I recommend starting your creatine intake 72 hours before the test for sure results.

Specific gravity measures the density of your urine and must be increased somehow because low specific gravity is almost a sure sign of dilution. Sugar and salt are known to increase specific gravity as are sports drinks such as Gatorade or PowerAde because of their electrolytes, sugar and salt content. For the brave, you might want to dump a tablespoon or so of salt and sugar into the sports drink for a little extra security.

To color your urine, you should take some B group vitamins and most multivitamin supplements contain these. Alternatively, you could use energy drinks that contain these vitamins such as Red Bull. Some multivitamins also contain zinc sulfate, which has been scientifically shown to mask THC metabolites. You can also find pure zinc sulfate supplements but don't go over 40mg if you decide to use it because it can be toxic. If you're going to use the dilution method, you'll need the following things:

- Creatine supplements or red meat

- Water

- Sports drinks (Gatorade, PowerAde)

- Cranberry juice

- Sugar

- Salt

- B complex vitamins

Now follow the steps below:

1) Begin taking creatine at least 24-72 hours before the test, either by eating a lot of red meat or taking creatine supplements. If you decide to use creatine supplements, you'll want to be taking at least 20g per day split into 4 phases of 5g each throughout the day. More specifically, you want at least 0.3g of creatine per kg of body weight.

2) On the day of the test, as soon as you wake up, go to the toilet and take a leak. Your first pee of the day contains the most THC metabolites.

3) Drink lots of water. On the days before the test this probably won't make much difference. But 2-3 hours before the test start by drinking 2, 8oz glasses of water. Then drink another 8oz every 15 minutes for the next hour. Within 1-2 hours you should be voiding clear, colorless urine every 20 minutes or so. Don't go overboard though—water toxicity is a real thing and can kill. In other words, cannabis is safer than water. Go figure.

4) After one hour, you can cut your water intake down to 3-4oz every 20-30 minutes to replace what you're losing through urination.

5) To increase specific gravity, drink a sports drink mixed with some salt and sugar about an hour before the test. By the way, feel free to replace the water entirely with Gatorade during this method. If you do this, there probably won't be much need to add salt and sugar to the drink. You might also want to drink cranberry juice to help flush the toxins into your urine and encourage higher creatinine levels.

6) 1-2 hours before the test, take the B complex vitamins to add some color to your urine. If they are time release, make sure you crush them before consuming. If you've decided to replace the water with Gatorade and cranberry juice this step may not be necessary since sports drinks often contain these vitamins already. Taking some zinc sulfate is also optional.

7) Take the drug test and provide a midstream urine sample.

This method has been proven to work even for heavy cannabis users. If they still say your sample is too dilute, despite your best efforts, just tell them you drink a lot of water. It's not as if drinking lots of water is anything out of the ordinary. You'll probably just have to come in at a later date for another test so try to schedule it as late as possible and don't dilute as much next time. If you find yourself in this situation and you're afraid of diluting again you may want to try this next method.

METHOD 3: SUBSTITUTION

Substitution is a 100% guaranteed way of passing a urine test if you do it right and is a walk in the park most of the time. But be warned— unlike the previous two methods this one can carry legal repercussions and harsh consequences if you are caught. If you get caught, you will have to carry out an observed test with someone watching you. This method involves taking in a substituted sample. That means either buying synthetic urine or taking in the urine of someone you know who is drug-free. If you are going to use someone else's urine to pass the test make sure that they haven't consumed any drugs and find out if they are on any type of prescription medications. Many prescription drugs contain things that would be otherwise illegal, such as opiates and amphetamines, and you could very well fail the drug test.

To do this method you'll need clean urine and an airtight container as a bare minimum. The container can be substituted for an unlubricated condom but you might want to rinse it with water first to remove any powder or latex smell. I should also warn you that condoms come with the added risk of potentially breaking open and revealing your secret, which is why I will stress the importance of practicing. It's pretty unlikely but it has happened to people before. Whatever you decide to use, it will need to hold at least 2oz of urine otherwise they may reject the sample for being too small. Light travel size shampoo bottles are perfect but if it previously stored shampoo make sure you wash it good. Fill your bottle with the urine and, while wearing tight underwear, store it down there to keep a nice temperature going. For men, store it between your crotch and under the testicles. Women can do the same thing but storing it in the vaginal cavity will maintain a more accurate temperature if it's not too uncomfortable.

You could tape a hand warmer to the outside of the container and place it between two pairs of underwear. Another option is to store it in a thermos with hot coffee, water, or other beverage. If the sample is too hot you can blow on it to cool it down while swishing it around and it will cool at a rate of about 1 degree every 30 seconds but don't cool it too much.

Maintaining a temperature of between 90-100 degrees Fahrenheit (body temperature) is absolutely crucial because a urine sample that is too cool will raise a huge red flag, as will a sample that is too hot. A thermometer isn't completely necessary but I strongly recommend you get one so that you can gauge the temperature of the sample before handing it to the collector. So buy a digital thermometer and make sure it doesn't make any noises or that the sound can be switched off. The temperature should stabilize at about 94 degrees if you've stored it correctly and can be slightly raised by crossing your legs and wedging it between your thighs for 10-15 minutes. Test cups often contain a temperature strip ranging from 90-100 anyway so you can see how warm your sample is before handing it in.

Do not use toilet or tap water to cool your sample. They sometimes color their toilet water blue to discourage anyone from using it and the collector often stands outside within earshot distance. If they hear you flushing the toilet or using tap water they might require you to resubmit a new sample. So do not flush and do not use the taps until you have given the collector your sample.

When you go to open the bottle containing the clean urine, do it very slowly and carefully. If the collector hears you opening or dropping something he's going to get suspicious and come knocking. If you're using a condom please be very careful as these have been known to drop everywhere except into the test cup when they are punctured incorrectly. Puncturing is a very risky and unpredictable way of emptying its contents. A better way would be to twist the condom, double it over itself, and then tightly hold it in place using a rubber band or wire tie. Then it's just a matter of untying everything and emptying the contents into the test cup.

You'll be asked to empty your pockets and take off your jacket before taking the test so, if you want to take in your thermometer or something like nail clippers for puncturing the condom, store them in your sock, underwear, or anywhere else you can get away with it. You can also put whatever you need in your pockets and empty everything except those items. It's unlikely you're going to get pat searched or anything—this isn't a federal prison. Just make sure that a thermometer isn't clearly bulging through your pockets and you'll be fine. I highly suggest that you practice substitution using warm water at home to get a "feel" for things and figure out the course of action you want to follow.

METHOD 4: TUBING

This method is essentially a variation of substitution but with an added twist. You'll basically be creating a device to store the clean urine sample that can also discharge it at the drug test and appear as if you are actually urinating. The device is designed for use by males but females could easily add their own twist to the method to make it work for them. This method is great for drug tests that are going to be observed. You're going to need the following materials:

- Latex balloon or condom

- Small fish tank tubing

- Aquarium airline tubing valve

- Rubber bands

- Tape

- Oral syringe

- Small hand warmers

- Coffee mug

- 2 pairs of boxer briefs

- Clean urine/synthetic urine

Now, there is a variation of this method which I will cover later. But for now, take a look at the steps below:

1) Rinse the latex balloon/ condom with some water and insert the fish tank tubing about 1 inch to halfway inside. Fasten it with a rubber band and secure it with the tape. You'll then need to cut the end of the tubing according to penis size, how far it will be down your boxer briefs, etc.

2) Inject urine into the tube with the syringe to fill your balloon with the clean sample and hold it in with the valve. If you don't have a valve, twist the balloon about 3 times and fold it.

3) Activate the hand warmer and place it into the coffee mug along with your device to maintain a good temperature. Now put on your 2 boxer briefs and go to the facility with your gear. You can use a thermometer to check the temperature on the way if you want to.

4) Boxer briefs have a large pocket underneath the testicle area. Place the hand warmer and the device here when no one is looking but make sure to do it on the outside of the first pair of boxers. Hand warmers can get very hot; this is why I recommend 2 pairs. Make sure the tube is facing upwards.

5) When you go to give the sample, either disengage the valve or reach in and unfold the balloon—it should untwist naturally. You can run the tube on the underside of your penis if someone is watching and they won't be able to see it. Now squeeze the balloon very gently and make the flow and sound look natural.

Remember that it's better if your sample is too warm rather than too cold because it can easily be cooled down. You should practice these steps at home as many times as you can using warm water. There is a variation of this method that is very good but also potentially uncomfortable and embarrassing. You'll need to use something like Vaseline to lubricate the balloon and insert it into your anus. Then use the syringe to fill the balloon with the urine. If you decide to do this, there won't be any need for hand warmers or a thermometer because the urine will be a perfect temperature the whole time but using a valve will almost certainly be necessary unless you kink the tube and fasten it in place somehow.

The urine sitting in the tube may be a different temperature than the urine in the balloon so you might want this to drop into the toilet before filling the cup. You can also increase the pressure of the stream by clenching. The key to this method is practice so that you know how to pull it off on the day of your drug test. And forgive me for continuing with my graphic descriptions, but for men there is a way of holding the tube underneath the penis and allowing it to trickle down the shaft so that it literally appears as if the urine is exiting the urethra.

Good luck my fellow stoner. Some of these methods may seem time-consuming, desperate, and embarrassing but do what you have to do.

URINE TESTS II: MYTHS AND FINAL TIPS

Try and find out as much information as you can about the place where you're taking the test beforehand because testing procedures can vary slightly from one place to the next. Ask around at local headshops, ask your friends and their friends, do an internet search on the facility or ask around on drug forums, etc. If you're really brave, you could actually call them and, using a bit of social engineering, find out what their testing procedures are.

If you're substituting, urine should be used within 8 hours. It can be refrigerated but if you don't need it for several days or more you should freeze it. Urine can be frozen in an airtight container for up to a year and still be good to use as a substitute after thawing with warm water. Another tip is to collect several bottles of your own urine during periods when you are THC-free and store it in a freezer so that you have clean samples to use at any time. Your urine must be between 90-100 degrees Fahrenheit so if you're using someone else's urine try to collect it as close to testing time as possible. Synthetic urine will need to be heated. You could always stop at a gas station on the way and ask to use their microwave if you forget.

However, there are a few problems with synthetic urine. Some of the products are just straight-up scams that won't help you but there are a few well-known brands that people swear by. Keep in mind that drug testing companies are always trying to develop ways of detecting synthetic urine. In addition, smelling urine is one way that some facilities use to determine the validity of the sample. This step isn't always followed for obvious reasons but synthetic urine is often scentless and if the collector does take a whiff of your sample you could get caught. In general, I find synthetic urine to be a waste of money if you can find someone willing to donate their own clean urine. Nevertheless, it can be a great thing to store in your car, toolbox, and so on if you know that random urine tests are used by your employer. You'll just have to heat it with a hand warmer for 20-

30 minutes. You can draw this time out by telling your employer that you don't have the urge to pee yet while you warm the urine.

There are prosthetic penises on the market that can be used to produce clean synthetic or substituted urine. Some people have gone so far as to recommend catheterization and filling your bladder with clean urine or even injections. To me, all of these seem to be overkill—especially that last one. Catheterization and bladder injections carry a high risk of infection and aren't worth the trouble. Prosthetic devices are now being checked for by some observers who will ask you to raise your shirt above the naval and lower your pants to mid-thigh level. If you're asked to do this you will almost certainly be caught because prosthetic penis devices are usually very bulky contraptions with straps, tubes, bags, and so on. They can be very expensive and are completely unnecessary if you follow the tubing method, which is much more discrete. If you do it right, you won't be caught using the tubing method if you're asked to pull up your shirt or pull down your pants.

If you're taking a physical exam at the same time as the drug test you may be asked to change into a gown at the beginning of the visit. So tell them that you really need to use the toilet and they might ask you to immediately provide the urine sample before taking you to the exam room.

Remember, looking sharp can go a long way. Don't show up for the test looking too rough and definitely don't show up wearing that cool shirt you have with a huge weed plant on the front of it. For the love of god, use some common sense! Authority figures won't admit that they're profiling but they often do. So if you somehow look like a drug user you're going to be treated like one. Sad but true.

Now let me talk a little bit about observed drug tests. There are two different types of observed drug tests: monitored collections and direct observations. Both of these are very uncommon and observers must be of the same gender. Observation is very rare in drug tests for purposes of employment unless you have been suspected of tampering with your urine sample or refused to empty your pockets. But it's not so unusual if you are on probation, for example. With monitored collections, a monitor will observe you from a distance either behind you or in very close proximity. They are there to ensure that no one else comes into the room; deter you from using unsecured water sources to tamper with your sample; or any of the other shenanigans people try to pull. With direct observations, they will either observe only the flow of urine or they will actually demand to see you physically deliver the urine.

They might use some type of screen to ensure that they are only observing the flow of urine or they may watch you through strategically placed mirrors, usually above the toilet or on the toilet lid. You can tell monitors or observers that you cannot pee with people watching and they might get tired of waiting and allow you to do it alone. Many people have successfully done this because having a shy bladder is indeed a very real problem. Otherwise, they might reschedule the drug test or give you a certain amount of time to drink water and wait until you can no longer hold it. At the very least, this could buy you some time to think of your next move. In some cases, you may be instructed to do a hair follicle test instead but this is very, very rare since these tests are much more expensive.

Substitution can be a difficult method to pull off if it's an observed test. However, I know a guy who was in prison for 8 years that successfully used his cell mate's urine to pass monitored drug tests. Sleight of hand, distraction, and believable excuses will go a long way. I recommend you practice the steps for the substitution and tubing method at home using water so that you can get a feel for the way you want to do it on the day of your test. Practice walking around with the hidden sample, practice getting the temperature right, practice opening the sample, practice putting the sample into a cup and so on and so forth. For monitored collections your chances of substituting are going to be higher than a directly observed drug test if you do it right. But you'll probably want to practice trying to mimic the sound of urinating using your bottle and opening it undetected. Simply pouring your sample into a cup is not going to look or sound very legit at all.

Myths and rumors concerning drug tests are not in short supply. Drug tests do not test for age, gender, race, favorite food or penis size. These were just myths that were perpetuated to discourage people from trying to substitute urine. Not only that, but it would be more expensive and time-consuming to do this and many facilities do not carry the equipment to do it. So don't go thinking you're anyone special and deserve to have an extra few hundred dollars burned on testing to see whether or not you're using your 5-year-old daughter's urine because they don't give a flying fig.

There are no legal repercussions for failing a drug test given by employers. You just won't get the position or you'll be fired. As a matter of fact, depending on the job and the employer, they might not even care if you were positive for marijuana. However, if you are on probation, in a custody battle, or you're in some other type of situation where you stand to lose a lot, it's just not worth it to consume marijuana because there may very well be consequences. When you have something this important on the line I strongly recommend that you stay clean.

Some people recommend using additives to pass a drug test. This involves urinating into the test cup and then adding something to it that supposedly masks drug metabolites. Additives used to work but this method has since gone the way of the cassette tape. You're almost guaranteed to get caught if you do this because drug testing methods and instruments have come a long way. These guys didn't spend thousands of dollars and years of their time to get a top-quality education and expensive testing gear only to be fooled by some pothead with a bottle of eye drops.

Detox products and herbal cleansing remedies are usually either completely useless or extremely unreliable. Some people swear by them and it probably wouldn't hurt to add it to your routine just to be safe but don't rely solely on these products to pass your test. Some of them tell you to consume the concoction while drinking lots of water and their ingredients often contain things such as creatine and vitamins. This just means that you would have chosen a very expensive way of completing the dilution method. If you have money to blow then it's completely up to you if you want to use these products. In my opinion, this money is better spent on buying some more weed. And please, don't try to drink bleach or any other wacky chemical to "detoxify"; you're probably just going to hurt yourself and fail the drug test.

If you're substituting, don't submit dog urine. Animal urine is rumored to work but it's just not worth the trouble trying to run around after your pet collecting their pee and there is a high risk of getting caught by the lab. The same goes for cat urine, rat urine, and monkey urine. Just don't bother.

SALIVA TESTS

The saliva test, also known as a swab test, is basically a joke and for this reason is not a very popular method when screening for drugs. That being said, it has become relatively common with some employers, particularly in Australia, where it is used as a random on-the-job drug test. And this is really their only benefit—they can be administered by the employer on-site. This makes swab testing useful as a random, post-accident, or return-to-duty drug test. Other benefits would be their ease of administration, convenience, cost-effectiveness, non-invasiveness, and fast results. In addition, it is difficult to tamper with a saliva test in the same way you could do with a urine test.

Not to worry though. The swab test is one of those rare cases where it is easier for a pothead to pass than a meth head. Meth can be detected 2-4 days after use while marijuana can generally be detected only for 12-24 hours after use and 3 days maximum. It's not uncommon for a heavy cannabis user to take a huge bong rip before sleeping and still pass their swab test the next morning. However, it would probably be unwise to do this.

Saliva testing is relatively new and the technology is not as developed as urine testing. This obviously works in your favor and despite its dubious track record you should still be aware of a few things. Swab testing technology is quite recent and companies are always going to be looking for ways to improve its effectiveness. It is doubtful that this will increase detection rates in any dramatic way but you should keep it in mind. Swab testing produces instantaneous results but it is sometimes sent to the lab for more accurate testing. However, this is generally more expensive and the detection time is no longer than the normal 1-3 days.

Saliva tests can come as a surprise to people who hadn't prepared for, or heard of, this particular method of testing and some businesses have made a habit of administering swab tests during job interviews. But there's no use in showing up to an interview with a bottle of your friend's piss between your butt-cheeks if they suddenly whip out a swab test that you hadn't prepared for. As they say, an ounce of prevention is worth a pound of cure. By taking a few simple preventative measures you should be able to pass this test with flying colors if it ever comes up.

Frequency of use is not so relevant when it comes to saliva tests. If a first-time cannabis user got high with a 40-year marijuana veteran yesterday, they are both just as likely to pass or fail a saliva drug test tomorrow. This is because swab tests actually test for recent intoxication/drug-use and the presence of actual THC rather than metabolites. This is why they are favored by certain employers who want to ensure that their workers aren't high on the job. Going to work high as a kite is a pretty stupid decision in the first place, especially in jobs where safety is a real concern. However, swab tests are notoriously easy to pass if you're not an idiot and know how to brush your teeth. There are saliva-cleansing products on the market that may be useful to carry around if your employer does random swab testing but they aren't completely necessary. You should stock up on the following items:

- Listerine strips/mints/gum

- Toothpaste

- Mouthwash

- Cigarettes (optional)

On the days before the test and the morning of the test, give your teeth a really good brush. You should also make a point of brushing your tongue, cheeks, and gum line. Do this at least twice a day, maybe even more. After brushing, use some good mouthwash to rinse. If they're also testing for alcohol, make sure you use a brand that doesn't contain alcohol. You might want to keep some mouthwash on you in a small bottle that can be used a few minutes before you take the test. Some like to use hydrogen peroxide to rinse their mouth as well but if you do this *do not* swallow it. I've never personally used peroxide so I can't vouch for its effectiveness or method of use.

For mints I recommend the Altoid brand. Otherwise you can use Listerine strips or strong chewing gum. People who have been caught with such things in their mouth prior to testing have been asked to remove them, drink water, and wait 15 minutes before they go in for the test. It is therefore assumed that mints and gum could possibly interfere with swab testing results. So if you're munching on Listerine strips before the test don't make it obvious around others and avoid boasting your fresh breath in front of them. Chewing on ice is also rumored to tip the odds in your favor. As for cigarettes, they supposedly help to mask THC remnants in the mouth so if you're a cigarette smoker you now have a good excuse to smoke.

If you get surprised with a swab test that you never prepared for there is one last strategy that can work. Hold the swab between your teeth while making sure that it does not touch the gums. Moisture from simply breathing may build up on the swab and allow for a negative test result. If you are asked to rub the swab back and forth between the lower cheeks and gum line, fake this movement by rubbing it on the teeth instead. After doing so you may be asked to leave it between the cheeks and gums for about 2 minutes. Again, you should hold it between the teeth so that any THC secretions from the gums cannot get onto the swab. Moreover, the swab should still be moist and appear to be a saliva sample.

It's not really known whether or not these measures actually fool the swab test or if the swab test is just a really bad method of detecting drugs. In any case, it won't hurt you to err on the side of caution. There is scientific evidence showing that THC does not enter saliva through diffusion from the bloodstream in the way that most other drugs do. On the one hand, this may be the reason that saliva tests are relatively easy for marijuana users to pass. On the other hand, this also means that you could show up positive by way of environmental contamination. In other words, even just sitting in a room where marijuana is being consumed can make you test positive and don't expect your employer to give a damn. One final thing, eating high-fat meals apparently helps to move drugs away from the mouth and into the digestive system. Since THC is fat soluble it wouldn't be unreasonable to assume that this does in fact help.

HAIR FOLLICLE TESTS

Ahhh, the dreaded hair follicle test. This is probably the most hated method of testing for drugs and with good reason—it is the most difficult test to cheat. Hair follicle tests are extremely difficult to tamper with or alter in any significant way. Moreover, your hair can betray your drug habits stretching back months or even years. Since hair grows at an average rate of approximately half an inch per month, this could theoretically mean that if your hair was 18 inches long you could find out which drugs you took 3 years ago if the ends were tested. Thankfully, most labs only require that you provide samples of the latest 1.5 inches of hair growth.

In general, you will be asked to provide approximately 40 strands of hair measuring about 1-1.5 inches in length, cut from the root. The non-root end is discarded. This is the standard procedure that most facilities follow and is enough to provide 60-90 days of drug history. If you haven't consumed any drugs for the past few months and they follow standard procedure you should be OK. The hair samples will almost always be taken from the head but if it's not long enough they will remove hair from your armpit, chest, or legs—and this is bad news. Hairs from these areas generally grow much slower and will contain a lot of information about your drug history within much smaller strands of hair. The sample is liquefied in a series of solvents to extract drug metabolites which are then analyzed in the lab.

However, there are a few things working in your favor. Firstly, hair tests are very expensive, which makes them a relatively rare method of pre-employment drug screening. If you're being asked to complete this kind of test I have to assume that you've applied for a fairly lucrative position. Secondly, THC and THC-COOH are lipophilic, meaning, as we discussed previously, they are attracted to fat. But hair has little to no fat content and is made mostly of protein. This means that THC and its metabolites are very weakly incorporated into hair; making hair tests a relatively unreliable way of testing for marijuana use. Other drugs such as cocaine and heroin are far more likely to be detected in hair than cannabis so if you are a marijuana-only drug user you have a greater chance of beating this test.

Another thing to keep in mind is that it's not uncommon for a false positive to show up on hair follicle tests. Police officers that are exposed to narcotics on a daily basis have been known to test positive as have children of drug consumers. So if you come up positive you might get away with using the excuse that some of your friends and family are drug users. This will be more believable if you're a very light marijuana consumer since the metabolite content in your hair is likely to be minimal. But heavy users would probably have a harder time trying to convince them of this.

One thing that frequently comes up in discussions about hair and THC is the idea that THC metabolites are incorporated into the hair through melanin. Unfortunately, if true, this means that people with dark hair are less likely to pass a hair follicle test because darker hair has higher concentrations of melanin. However, scientific testing has not been able to definitively confirm this as true. Nevertheless, if this theory does happen to be correct, this could be the reason that bleaching hair is claimed to help beat a hair test because melanin is oxidized into a colorless compound. This leads us to our first method.

METHOD 1: BLEACHING
If you decide to do this, you will need the following:

- Olive oil

- Shower cap

- Shampoo (Aloe Rid/Zydot/Toxin Wash recommended)

- 40 volume peroxide bleach kit

- (optional) Hair dye

Once you have these items follow this process:

1) Use 1 or 2 tablespoons of olive oil (depending on hair length) and work it into the hair until it's saturated. Place a shower cap on your head and let it sit for 30 minutes to an hour. This step isn't completely necessary but olive oil works great as a deep conditioner and some of the THC metabolites may bind with the oil. Rinse thoroughly.

2) Wash and scrub your hair with some good shampoo. I would recommend Aloe Rid shampoo. NORML once suggested using this brand before a hair follicle test and many have reported good results just using this alone. Other recommended brands have been Zydot and Toxin Wash. Place the shower cap back on your head and let it sit in your hair for a while (30 minutes if you're paranoid—keep scrubbing the whole 30 minutes if you're *really* paranoid). Rinse thoroughly.

3) Get a 40 volume peroxide bleach kit and bleach the hell out of your hair. Avoid getting it on your skin because it burns. You could buy all of the necessary ingredients and create your own mixture if you wanted to. Alternatively, get this done professionally by someone who actually knows what they're doing. I won't cover all of the necessary steps to bleach your hair because that's an art unto itself depending on the length of your hair but you can find a zillion guides on how to do it on the internet. Let the bleach soak through until you're satisfied or repeat this step as necessary and rinse well with cold water.

4) Dye your hair back to your original color if you want to and then give your hair a good rinse. You can find out how to do this with a 2 second Google search if you're unsure. Again, getting this done by a pro will make things much easier.

5) Repeat step 2 and rinse.

6) Repeat step 1 and rinse.

METHOD 2: THE MACCUJO METHOD

Next to bleaching, the second most popular method for passing a hair test is known as the MacCujo method. Back in 2003, an internet forum poster going by the name "MacCujo" posted the method he was using to pass hair tests. This person claims to have been shown these steps by a friend who worked in a testing lab. Since then, many people have reported success using this method but I must warn you—this is going to burn. Make sure you have a towel handy to wipe up anything that drips. You could also apply Vaseline around the forehead, ear and neck areas before doing this so that the stinging sensation is minimized. Wearing goggles might also be a good idea because you don't want any of this getting into your eyes. Your hair will feel really terrible after doing this so apply some olive oil afterwards. You will need:

- Vinegar

- Clean and Clear

- Laundry detergent

- Shampoo (Aloe Rid/Neutrogina TSal/Zydot/Toxin Wash)

- Olive oil

- Shower cap

This method involves the following:

1) Soak hair in vinegar for 10-30 minutes while wearing a shower cap. Wipe anything that drips. Try to find apple cider vinegar for this step.

2) Massage Clean and Clear into the hair to mix it with the vinegar. This product is for acne and should be pink with 2% salicylic acid. This supposedly cleans metabolites after the vinegar opens the pores. Wear the shower cap and leave it in for another 30 minutes if you can withstand the burning.

3) Rinse your hair while scrubbing it with laundry detergent. Most variations of this method insist on using the brand Tide. I'm not sure if this matters or not but I may be missing something. You can do this for up to 30 minutes but rinse everything out when you're finished.

4) Now scrub your hair with the shampoo and rinse. Again, you can do this for up to 30 minutes if you think it will help.

5) Your hair will feel pretty terrible at this point so use some olive oil as a conditioner and then rinse it out.

Be warned, you might reek of vinegar after doing this process and that's going to raise a huge red flag when you go for the test. If you have this problem, you may want to use some hair gel, hair spray, or some other type of hair product that will mask the smell and spray your body with deodorant. You can repeat the MacCujo Method several times leading up to the drug test if you so desire. Personally, I've never used this method before and I'm skeptical of its effectiveness but it has worked for others.

Another method to use would be applying hair relaxer, rinsing with shampoo, and then applying a moisturizing conditioner. Applying hair relaxer has been scientifically proven to reduce the presence of drug metabolites because it breaks down the chemical bonds of the hair. It is typically used for perms and hair straightening. However, I will not be covering the steps for this method because I've never done it myself and I strongly recommend you get it performed by a professional. Applying hair relaxer incorrectly can lead to very damaged hair and even permanent hair loss so please do your research if you're going to do this.

If you have the time, stay clean for 2 weeks before using any of these methods because hair can take a while to expose itself above the scalp. This means that even if you've stopped smoking, hair with THC-COOH content could take 1-2 weeks to grow above the scalp. So if you've worked hard to treat your hair with one of these methods you may have wasted your time if the test isn't for another week or two.

Your other option is to treat your hair as close to the testing day as possible. I advise that you do this anyway because these methods can be damaging for your hair and you don't want to be doing it for weeks on end.

Note that none of these methods have been confirmed scientifically to help you beat a hair follicle drug test. These are simply the two most popular methods that cannabis users have claimed worked for them. It's a lengthy process, your head might burn, and you could ruin your hair if you aren't careful. You'll just have to suck it up if you're this desperate. As with the saliva test, it is difficult to tell whether or not these methods actually help or if the hair follicle test has an unpredictable detection rate for marijuana.

In the worst case scenario, you could shave every inch of hair on your body or to the point where no testable sample can be taken. I would recommend that you shave everything except your head anyway so that they're forced to take samples from your head if they ever try to get samples from elsewhere. For women this shouldn't be a problem. If you're a guy, you could claim you're an athlete of some sort if they ask about it but this excuse is obviously going to be a tad unbelievable if you're clocking in at something like 200 pounds of mostly fat so use your imagination.

However, you should be aware that some facilities have stated that if you have no hair to collect it will be considered a refusal to test. In this case, you could ask your employer about the possibility of a retest within several weeks when your hair grows back. You could use a product that promotes hair growth to make the time go faster. Don't smoke anything during this period and you'll have a clean hair sample to provide but remember to take into account what I said above about drug-affected hair taking up to 2 weeks to grow above the scalp. Some people have reported that they were simply asked by their employer to take a urine test instead when they didn't have enough hair to test. In this case, refer to the chapters on urine testing.

One final note, if you haven't been smoking for a while you could easily just get your hair trimmed down to a level where no THC metabolites will be present in your hair. This usually isn't necessary since they only take the latest 1-1.5 inches of growth to test your past 3 month drug history. But if you can do it then do it and don't take any risks. Make sure not to cut it too short, especially if you haven't cut any body hair, otherwise they'll start taking samples from your armpits, legs, or chest and you could fail the test despite being marijuana-free for several months.

BLOOD AND SWEAT TESTS

Blood tests are very, very rare because they are extremely invasive and difficult to administer. Usually, blood tests are only used to detect recent drug use by searching for the presence of actual THC. Using a blood test to detect metabolites would generally be a waste of money because urine and hair follicle tests can do a much better job of this and at a cheaper price. I have never heard of anyone having to take a blood test for purposes of employment. Blood tests are typically only used in the investigation of accidents, injuries, and DUIs to accurately determine whether or not the subject was impaired at the time. Some insurance companies may require blood samples when assessing financial risk.

Cannabis can only be detected in blood for around 1-3 days and up to a month if they are looking for metabolites. Almost always they will be testing only for the presence of THC in the blood because there are much better ways to detect the metabolites. If you have to take a blood test you're pretty much screwed because they are the most accurate test out there and next to impossible to fool. Moreover, in the case of a DUI or an accident you'll likely be tested within a few hours with no prep time. If you've been given prior warning about a blood test then steer clear of marijuana for 24-48 hours at the least and you should be fine. I've heard that drinking a lot of energy drinks such as Red Bull can help you pass a blood test but I wouldn't bet my life on it.

As for sweat tests, these consist of a sweat patch that is worn for an extended period of time, usually a week or so. The sweat patch consists of a gauze pad covered with something similar to a Band-Aid and sticks tightly to the skin. Isopropyl alcohol is applied to the area before application, typically on the upper arm. The gauze pad is sent to a lab for analysis after the subject has worn the patch for the allotted time period.

Sweat patches are primarily used on prisoners, military personnel and people on probation or parole. According to some research that has been done, sweat patches will not detect marijuana in most people if they have been clean for at least a week but chronic users can still test positive for up to 4 weeks. However, sweat patches are notorious for false positive results because they can be contaminated so easily. Sweat patches can be contaminated by the person applying or removing the patch if they have drug residue on their hands or gloves. It is also thought that sweating can encourage environmental contamination in a variety of ways. This can include being in close proximity to drug users or even accidental transferring of cocaine residue found on currency.

Nevertheless, they have an unreliable detection rate for marijuana because cannabinoids eliminated from the body through sweat have very low concentrations. Heavy users are detected more frequently than light users. You should be warned that excessive sweating can result in the patch losing its adhesiveness and you will be automatically declared positive for suspected tampering.

There is one method that has been claimed to work for cheating a sweat patch drug test. After they apply the patch you should immediately use a hair dryer to heat the adhesive and, with clean hands, pull it back slightly. Then take a piece of aluminum foil or something of the sort to wedge between the patch and your skin. Before you go to have the patch removed, take out the foil and apply some adhesive glue to seal the patch again. Please be careful doing this because you will be failed for tampering if you do a slipshod job. If you're going to consume marijuana throughout the period you are wearing the patch, you should probably cover it with something as an extra precaution to prevent external contamination from smoke or residue.

CONCLUSION

This book has given you all the information, strategies, and methods you could ever want or need to pass any type of marijuana drug test. But you have to be the one to take action—an ounce of prevention is worth a pound of cure. As a matter of fact, an ounce of prevention could be the difference between your next pound of marijuana and 200 pounds of your new cell mate waiting for you to bend over.

Allow me to recap the two most important points that you must follow before taking a drug test. Firstly, stop consuming marijuana—I know it sucks but if you cannot do that then perhaps you have other problems to deal with. Secondly, practice the methods. Practice is particularly essential for passing a urine test because you want be sure that the sample maintains a good temperature and you need to have a good understanding of the steps that you'll have to go through on the day. Foiling an otherwise good plan is going to cost you a lot more than the preparation and practice you should have put in.

Having said all of that, you should also take into account other factors that are going to affect your chances of passing a test, which can vary from person to person. These factors include things such as weight, amount of exercise, frequency of cannabis use, type of test, and the type of cannabis preparation you have been consuming. This might also affect the type of method you wish to use. For example, a very light marijuana consumer may choose to go with exercise or dilution rather than substitution, and vice versa. I would recommend you practice and experiment with home drug tests to see what works for you.

Thank you again for getting this book. Remember, knowledge is power. If the information in this book was enjoyable or helpful in any way, please take the time to share your thoughts and post a review on Amazon.

ABOUT THE AUTHOR

Simon Stone is an advocate for the complete legalization of marijuana and psychedelics and is a firm supporter for ending the War on Drugs. He has a degree in political science and loves travelling to broaden his mind. Simon is married with two children and writes on a variety of subjects that interest him. His motto is, "Question everything and follow reason."

If you wish to contact Simon or discuss this book, please visit the official Pryde Publishing social media pages:

Facebook: facebook.com/PrydePublishing

Twitter: twitter.com/PrydePublishing.